The Painless Period Guide

A Guide To Accessing The Power Of Your Menstrual Cycle

Eat the Right Nutrients for Hormone Balance
Get Rid of Bloating, Nausea, and Pain
Sleep Through the Night Without Waking from Cramps
Learn Self-Care Rituals
Get Answers Beyond the Pill!

Selin Bilgin

B.A, C.H.N. Certified in Holistic Nutrition,
Women's Wellness Educator

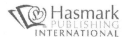
Hasmark
PUBLISHING
INTERNATIONAL

Editor:
Brad Green
brad@hasmarkpublishing.com

Interior layout:
Amit Dey amit@hasmarkpublishing.com

Cover design:
HedgehogIndustries

ISBN 13: 978-1-989756-97-3
ISBN 10: 1989756972

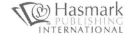

Note to the Reader

The information in this book is not intended or implied to be a substitute for professional medical advice, diagnosis, or treatment. All content, including texts, graphics, images, and other information contained in this book is for general information purposes only.

Bilgin Holdings Ltd. and Luscious Living make no representation and assume no responsibility for the accuracy of information contained in this book, and such information is subject to change.

You are encouraged to verify any information obtained from this book by exploring other sources, and discuss any and all information regarding medical conditions or treatments with your physician.

NEVER DISREGARD PROFESSIONAL MEDICAL ADVICE OR DELAY SEEKING MEDICAL TREATMENT BECAUSE OF SOMETHING YOU HAVE READ IN THIS BOOK.

Bilgin Holdings Ltd. and Luscious Living do not recommend, endorse, or make any representation about the efficacy, appropriateness, or suitability of any specific tests, products, procedures, treatments, services, opinions, healthcare providers, or other information that may be contained in this book.

BILGIN HOLDINGS LTD. AND LUSCIOUS LIVING ARE NOT RESPONSIBLE OR LIABLE FOR ANY ADVICE, COURSE OF TREATMENT, DIAGNOSIS, OR ANY OTHER INFORMATION THAT YOU OBTAIN THROUGH THIS BOOK

Table of Contents

Dedication

This book is dedicated to the women of the world.
May we rise together.

Acknowledgments

As a young girl, there was nothing more I loved in the world than books. Not much has changed.

As first grader Selin, you could find me writing fantasy books about mythical creatures, all bound with a cover made of cardboard paper and markers. While this book does not feature any fanciful creatures, my hope is that it will guide you on your journey in realizing your power, as well understanding your menstrual health too. My aim is to assist you in alleviating potentially one of the most frustrating and painful aspects of a woman's experience …our period!

Many of us have the experience of our menstruation being an embarrassing, uncomfortable, frustrating, debilitating, or even downright disgusting and unfortunate incident. I get it. I've been there. Perhaps this book will have you not just "put up" with your menstrual cycle, but to actually know your body, and love yourself!

This book could not have been completed without some of the most important people in my life.

To my parents, Serdar and Yasemin Bilgin, who raised me with love. It was through your affection for each other that I learned what true love really is. I could not have asked for better parents. Rest in Peace, dad. I love you forever.

To Peggy McColl, a *New York Times* best-selling author who gently nudged me through the process by asking: *When is your book coming out?* Peggy, thank you, thank you, thank you!

To my best friends, Stephanie, Vivian, Andrea, and Jillian, who have shown me generosity, love, and support from the beginning. Thank you for being true friends.

To Barbara, at HedgehogIndustries on Etsy, who kindly created the most beautiful book cover illustration that I could have ever asked for. Thank you!

Finally, to the love of my life, and number one supporter, Eric Webb. Thank you for being the man that you are. Thank you for your endless encouragement, profound love, and PATIENCE! I love you beyond words.

The premenstrual phase is therefore a time when we have greater access to our magic—our ability to recognize and transform the more difficult and painful areas of our lives. Premenstrually, we are quite naturally more in tune with what is most meaningful in our lives. We're more apt to cry—but our tears are always related to something that holds meaning for us. Years of personal and clinical experience have taught me that the painful or uncomfortable issues that arise premenstrually are always real and must be addressed.

—Dr. Christiane Northup

Introduction

Hi! I'm pretty darn excited that you're here. I hope you make yourself comfortable and nourished as much as possible while reading this book.

My name is Selin Bilgin (pronounced as *Celine*) and I am a speaker, a Certified Holistic Nutrition Consultant™, and a women's health educator.

Whether you are here because you have awful periods yourself and desire relief, you are someone who would love to understand your own body better, you have been missing periods, you do not have a uterus anymore, or anything else I may not have mentioned; my intention is that all of you are welcome here.

I wrote this book for you. My vision and mission is to have a seriously sweet impact on women around the planet so that they may live their most radiant and vibrant lives, beginning with their health. I believe that when women are empowered...the world is empowered.

As women, we have a magical ability to uplift the people around us (and far beyond!) when *we* too are uplifted, empowered and feeling vibrant from the inside out. When we live in alignment with our spirit and heart, a healthy body follows suit. When we feed our mind, body, and spirit with thoughts, activities and environments that are nourishing, we are then better able to nourish ourselves, our planet and its people as well, and with greater ease and joy. This is true regardless of whether your role is that of a mother, a student, a wife, a teacher, or the CEO of a Fortune 500 company.

This book focuses primarily around PMS pain and menstrual health. I do not go into detail about other hormonal challenges, such as PCOS and endometriosis, although the concepts in this book can be considered foundational. I am confident that you will find this information helpful.

Here's a bold statement: You *can* have a painless period!

Yet we have been led to believe that it's normal.

You do not need to have a painful period; in fact, you can actually learn to *love* your period..

If you spend two weeks out of every four suffering with PMS or menstruation (or even another minute, sis!) it doesn't have to be this way. My clients and myself are living examples of this truth.

My journey of wellness was built through struggle (perhaps that is where good stories and growth comes from). By the time I was in eighth grade, I had a condition called hyperhidrosis (excessive sweating) because I was so anxious (and highly embarrassed at that point I may add). As for my period, I used to rely on painkillers in order to even get through my periods and would wake up at night from cramping. I felt "gross", fatigued and bloated when I was on my cycle. I had terrible hormonal acne, and took a popular (and pricey) pharmaceutical drug to help (it didn't). By sixteen, I was on sleeping pills in order to sleep at night (which didn't help either) and had already contemplated ending my life several times. By the time I was twenty-two, I was officially bulimic. When I stopped hurting myself in that way, I was binge eating and addicted to food, and had gained over forty pounds in a single year. I didn't leave the house from the shame I had around it. Then, after a trip to Italy, I found myself having four periods in ONE month!

After that, I had two periods in a single month for a year. You will find out how I overcame that in this book, using the nutrition and lifestyle principles that I now teach.

Why do I share that?

Girl, if I can overcome ALL of this, and to continue to become the most vibrant and flourishing version of myself (mentally, spiritually and physically) **you can too**. I am a masterpiece in progress, and **so are you.**

Again, this book is all about YOU! Please enjoy it.

You can also connect with me on Instagram @_LusciousLiving_ and listen to the Luscious Living podcast on iTunes, Spotify, or Stitcher for more inspiration and information!

Please note that throughout this book you may find ideas that you love, and others that don't resonate. Please take what works for you, and leave the rest. Ultimately, you are the boss of your own body!

In love and service,

Selin Bilgin

Chapter 1

Life Design 101

You are a powerful creator.

Your consistent words, thoughts, and actions are all co-creating the life that you are living today...as well as the life that you will live tomorrow, and for years to come.

How?

Think about it. Look around you.

Everything that you see at first was nothing more than a thought. The planter, the painting, the meal, everything. Someone (or you) thought:

> *I need something to hold this plant. This would look nice here.*
>
> *I'm hungry.*

All things first spring from the mind. Then, as Hermetic Principles states that every cause has its effect; every effect has its cause, or Newton's third law of motion states that for every action there is an equal and opposite reaction...from that thought, our mind then communicates with our body, creating a feeling.

Our feelings are powerful indicators of what me may be thinking consciously, or subconsciously. Below is an example of how thoughts impact actions:

Alarm Rings

Person number one: "Wow, it's so cozy and warm in bed. I don't feel like getting up right now … but I'm going to get up anyway! I'm going to get up, and go kick butt today!"

Gets out of bed, goes for a run, eats breakfast, gets ready for work, has a great day

Or:

Alarm rings

Person number two: "Ughhhhh not again. Five more minutes. I am SO not a morning person…" (*presses snooze on the alarm*) "Ahhhh, I slept in again! I don't even have time to eat breakfast. Where the heck are my keys?! I'm going to be late - again!"

(I've been both scenarios by the way). Can you see how, even in a simple scenario like this, it is our **thoughts** that lead to our action? Many times, our thoughts and actions are so habitual that we don't even spend our conscious thoughts thinking about it.

The important thing to remember is that in order to change our results, we must first begin to make changes from the inside out. Wait, isn't this a book about period health!? Yes darling, and, in order to get to that space of feeling in sync, we must begin at the level of our thoughts and mindset.

So, how do you do that? It all begins with creating a vision.

Vision Crafting

This could be one of the most important things that you do: creating the vision of the woman you desire to be.

To start, grab a pen and paper (or electronic document), your favorite drink, and begin to write.

Here are some steps to help you begin:

Step One: Define and Describe

Define the version of you that you dream of being. It could be you in a month, or 6 months, or 5 years from now. I want you to do this by describing, your ideal you...:

What is her ideal morning ritual? What time does she go to sleep, and what time does she wake up? What kinds of foods does she enjoy? What does her perfect work day and weekend look like? How does she dress and adorn herself? What kinds of accessories, hairstyles, or makeup does she invest in? What does she do for work? How does she move her body? What does her home look like? Is she organized? What do her finances look like?

How does she feel about herself and others? About other women? What does she do to treat herself, or to please herself? What kinds of rituals does she honour? How does she comfort herself when she is sad, disappointed or feeling lonely?

What does she need to start letting go of? (Thoughts, people, expenses?) What would she like to cultivate more of?

If you struggle with any ongoing health conditions or symptoms: Who would she be if she no longer struggled with her current health challenges? What would she be thinking about or doing instead? What would her life look like instead?

Step Two: Envision and Create

Be sure to go back and read those things you wrote about yourself on a daily basis. You may want to print it too! It's important to tap into the FEELING of this woman. Then I'd like for you to write out tangible actions you would need to create in order to achieve these ideals. Make a list and put it in your calendar. Small steps build momentum.

How would you be thinking and acting if you already WERE that woman?

What else can you do to anchor this in? (Vision boards, affirmations, songs, etc?) Once you begin to do this, you will be astonished at how quickly these things begin to manifest themselves in your life. You will begin to act as if you already are the woman that you desire to be, and soon enough, you will be her!

Affirmations and Mantras

We are both spiritual *and* physical beings.

While we will focus on specific nutrients and body-related actions in this book, I also want to quickly touch on the powerful impact that affirmations or mantras can have on your journey.

To become the women that we desire to be and support ourselves from the inside out, we must first affirm our own power to ourselves.

With my nutrition practice, I hear a lot of women (and I am not perfect at this!) say:

"I should…"

"She, or he, or they should…"

"I don't know…"

"I wish…"

"I will try..."

"I will never..."

"I have to..."

Instead, begin to affirm by using phrases that are more empowering to you, such as:

"I choose to..."

"I get to..."

"I will..."

"I commit to..."

"I will figure out how to..."

"I don't know now, but I will find out..."

"I'm grateful to, or grateful for..."

Begin to sense how different the statements above feel in comparison to the previous ones. The first list completely takes the power out of you, and places it elsewhere. What happens when we place the power outside of ourselves? We become victims. If we become victims, we cannot change our circumstances and are therefore powerless. We get to be right about our failures and about not being good enough. Whereas, if we affirm our power (not in an egotistical way, but rather, through the innate spiritual power that is in us all) and take 100% responsibility for our lives, then can we actively seek and attract an abundance of opportunities and solutions.

So remember, you can, and you must tell yourself that you can.

With that as a reminder, when it comes to PMS—and in life in general— you have the power!

Affirm your power and strength, take action, and go out there and be the badass that you know you are!

Chapter 2

Menses: A Brief History and the Four Phases of Your Cycle

Let's get into it, shall we!

As you have by now realized, your menstrual cycle runs on a continuous loop from your first period until you hit menopause, stalled only by the occasional baby-making, if you so choose (*bow chicka wow-wowwww*).

Unlike what is currently understood by most people, menstruation was originally considered a sacred process that equipped women with intuitive powers and wisdom. As you now know, menstruation is often regarded as something disgusting, painful or useless. This is a sad understanding, and it's not true.

My aim with this book is that you will learn to love your moon time, that you will get in tune with your cycle and harness the power that is within you.

Papyrus, Buffalo Skin, and The Red Tent

When we realize the process of menstruation is so deeply connected to our spiritual energies, it opens up new pathways for healing and living life in sync with nature. You become amazed at yourself!

It is undeniable that we live in the best of times. We can book an Airbnb in Tokyo, order a pizza in Milan, and pay bills at home, all while soaking in the bathtub with sparkly purple bath bomb fizzing away. On the menstrual side of things, we can have tampons delivered straight to our door or have reliable reusable menstrual products available at the touch of a finger. We still have further to go, but the truth is that most women in history would not recognize the pads and tampons we use today, which only became mainstream in the 1960s and 70s.

According to the book, *Flow: The Cultural Story of Menstruation* by Elissa Stein and Susan Kim, women in Egypt used papyrus as tampons. In ancient Greece and Rome, women created tampons by wrapping lint around wood. In ancient Japan, women used paper to absorb blood, while the Native Americans made pads out of moss and buffalo skin. These were the first "all natural" products. Wow!

The Red Tent

This is one of my favorite notions of menstrual history. In pre-modern cultures, women would gather together in a hut and bleed directly onto the ground. Then, after their bleed, they would come back to the tribe with wisdom to share. The female cycle was revered and worshipped in ancient cultures by men and women for its life-bearing ability. Consequently, women honored their bodies once a month; they lived life at a different pace, without responsibility, while getting plenty of rest. Sounds like a far, far away time doesn't it?!

Nowadays, many women do not have the luxury of resting during our cycle, let alone during regular times. Many of us wear many different hats. We are full-time (or single) mothers, we are students, we are executives; we are a myriad of roles, and we often run ourselves thin. In alignment with that reality, many of us view our period as an inconvenience, and many of us experience trouble during this time (cramping, bloating, nausea, mood swings, acne).

See, I used to think my menstrual cycle was disgusting and embarrassing. My heart goes out to my younger self and younger period now for even thinking that. I'm curious: how do you view it? Is it inconvenient? Beautiful? Is it a time for rest? Our mind is powerful, and I believe we are constantly creating as we speak. I know it may be an incredibly frustrating and painful experience for some, but I encourage you to identify at least one thing it allows you to experience. For example, are you needing more alone time, and being on your period actually provides you with the opportunity to spend time with yourself? Maybe you get to leave work early, or completely miss work, knowing deep down that you didn't want to be there anyway, and that it may be time to create something new? I invite you to consider this question deeply.

Significance of Each Phase in the Cycle

I'd like to teach you about your four phases. When you begin to live in tune with your feminine cycle, you will begin to understand and love your body. You will be more aware of what your body needs and desires. No longer should you feel guilty about having less energy during your luteal phase, or feeling inconsistent in your workouts from one week to the next. I speak from personal experience!

Your monthly cycle consists of four phases: menstrual, follicular, ovulatory, and luteal. You can learn to optimize each phase and become the woman that you desire to be.

Week 1: Menstrual Phase (Days 1-7)

This phase begins on the first day of bleeding and is considered your *internal winter*. Think of this as the process of the cleansing and removal of negative thoughts, emotions, and toxins. Our natural biological cleansing is accompanied by a psychological cleansing. You may notice that within the first few days of your period (once your periods become enjoyable!) you may feel an urge to suddenly clean or reorganize your home. This is the time when women feel the need to go inward, to be silent and contemplative. I personally like to journal, meditate and pull cards more around this time. You will naturally experience a decrease in energy and hormone levels, and an increase in appetite. So, give yourself permission to nurture yourself! This is the time to eat nourishing foods, listen to your hunger, and stay warm.

This is also the ideal time to have low-intensity movement such as Pilates, yin yoga, or taking long walks.

Here are some suggested activities: journaling (we are highly intuitive at this time), meditating, participating in a virtual or in-person sound bath, chanting, breathwork, baking, organizing, and napping.

If you are going to be sexually active during this time, please be sure to use lubrication. Your hormones are at their lowest point, so estrogen is not providing as much natural lubrication.

Week 2: Follicular Phase (Days 7-14)

This is the phase that is aligned with your *inner spring*. The steady increase in estrogen boosts your brain's serotonin levels, leading to an increase in energy, enthusiasm, and a more upbeat feeling overall. Yay! This phase is considered ideal for kicking off new projects or creative work, and for focusing more on fresh, lightly steamed foods.

For physical movement and life in general during this phase, think *new* or fresh energy! New goals, new workouts, new ideas. If you've been considering taking a belly dancing or jujitsu class, now is the perfect time to go for it! Think of new ingredients, new recipes, new date ideas, or new activities to do with your kids during this inner spring.

Week 3: Ovulation Phase (Days 14 – 21)

This is your inner summer, babe! The ovulation phase is the time when women are more physically attractive compared to other days (You're always hot. Due to the increase of your sex hormones, it simply adds a little more spice to your step!), and are more attracted to others.

During this phase, our skin, hair, and eyes are glowing; thank you Estrogen! This is the time in our cycle when we need to be connecting, networking and going out to that new museum or bar.

This is the time to focus more on raw, fresh foods, and go all out in our high intensity workouts! (If you do have a hormone imbalance - I would caution you on doing high intensity workouts until that is balanced in order to balance cortisol. You will learn more about this hormone and estrogen dominance later.) Ladies, ovulation is a sign of health (US National Library of Medicine), and should not be dismissed. Birth control pills and other oral contraceptives stop ovulation (if there is no egg released, there is nothing for sperm to fertilize and, therefore, no pregnancy.) Lara Briden, the author of *The Period Repair Manual,* states: "If you are not thinking about ovulation, you are not thinking about your health." I agree. I would strongly consider whether or not birth control pills are a beneficial option for your long term future. This is also the best time to get pregnant if you are trying!

(Side note: How can you tell if you are ovulating? And what if you are not ovulating at all?)

Six Signs of Ovulation:

1. Cervical Mucus - Check your underwear! Your mucus will be similar to an egg white in. Cervical mucus serves the purpose of accepting, filtering, preparing, and conveying sperms on their journey to the egg. Oh how amazing our body is.

2. Increased Libido - Read above as your inner summer. This is the body's natural reaction to ovulation. Ow ow!

3. Elevated Basal Body Temperature - After 24 hours after the egg's release, your temperature rises and stays up for several days. Before ovulation, a woman's temperature averages between 36.1°C (97°F) and 36.4°C (97.5°F). After ovulation, it rises to 36.4°C (97.6°F) to 37°C (98.6°F) (Health Link BC).

4. Cervical Position - Throughout a cycle, the cervix, located at the end of the "tunnel" in the vagina, changes position. Outside of the fertile window, the cervix is lower, harder, and more closed. Prior to ovulation, the cervix moves higher and becomes softer and more open. Feel for yourself!

5. Ovulation Pain - A bit of cramping may happen, which may be an egg breaking free from the ovary during ovulation.

2 main reasons why you may not be ovulating (and then some more)

Hormonal birth control

As mentioned above, most types of hormonal contraception work by switching off ovulation. You may experience something called "break-through bleeding" which is not a real menstrual cycle!

Polycystic ovary syndrome (PCOS)

Polycystic ovary syndrome (PCOS) is a hormonal condition typically marked by elevated testosterone, insulin and inflammation. I work with a lot of women with PCOS so please feel free to reach out.

Undereating

Hypothalamic amenorrhea (HA) is the loss of periods due to undereating or under eating carbohydrates. Other possible causes include thyroid disease, high prolactin, gluten sensitivity, zinc deficiency, a strict vegan diet, and certain medications.

Week 4: Luteal (Days 21 – 28)

Think of this as your *inner fall* or *autumn*. During this time, you will feel a desire to move inward and slow down. What's neat is that research shows greater activity in the right hemisphere of the brain (the part associated with intuitive knowing) during weeks three and four of your cycle! So, trust your intuition, and give it extra close attention during the second half of your cycle. *This is where most women start to experience symptoms of PMS* (though with this guide, you'll be smooth sailing!)

Begin to eat more grounding, warming foods, and incorporate more complex carbs and fiber into your diet. You will start to become more hungry and require a slower pace than you did in your follicular or ovulatory phase. This is a phase where I would like for you to optimize first to begin to see noticeable changes. I will speak later about this again in the book, though if you experience breast tenderness for example on your period, start to increase your vitamin E rich foods and/or supplementation at this time. If you experience cramps, begin to increase your omega's and magnesium rich foods and/or supplementation, and decrease or eliminate common triggers such as dairy, gluten, soy and corn. If you are a chocolate lover like me, your body is typically asking for more magnesium, so see what a magnesium bath, magnesium supplementation, and raw cacao does for you. Once you begin to track your cycle, you will begin to notice these subtle (or not so subtle) shifts. If you can, I encourage you to take more time for yourself at this time. I know some of you reading this may have kids, and even thirty minutes to an hour will help immensely (and get your partner, in-laws, friends and/or babysitter on board!). Whether you take this time to rest, or create, it will help with any low moods or irritability.

The luteal phase also is the best time to focus on strength training; body weights, pilates, barre, or other strength training exercises rather than your long runs or boxing class like in your luteal phase. This is also the best time to wrap up projects, ideas, and tie up any loose ends at work and at home.

The Full Circle:

So how do you begin to implement these changes into your life?

As of now, we do not live in a world that yet supports living in tune with our feminine phases, so there is no need to be "perfect" with this and you can do the best you can. Listen to your body.

I recommend first and foremost, using an app, or if you're like me, using your paper calendar to mark which day of the week you are in, and begin to map it out from there. I like to make a red dot on each day of my menstrual cycle. I find it incredibly helpful to track where I am, and to better understand my needs and desires. I hope you now release any guilt about feeling more fatigued, not wanting to socialize, coming up with new ideas at work, and/or wanting to go for a run instead of lifting weights for example. You are a different woman in different phases!

Discussion Topics:

1. Do you currently track the phases of your cycle? Is that something you think would be beneficial?

2. Ask yourself: What kind of physical movement am I craving right now? Does my body need to eat warmer foods, or more fresh and raw foods?

3. Journal about the things you think you may need during your PMS symptoms. For example, you've been in a constant rush all month, and being on your period with intense symptoms finally gives you a reason to rest. Or, perhaps you want to start meal prepping, but you find yourself in a vicious cycle of ordering out, knowing that isn't how you want to spend your hard-earned money.

Action Steps:

1. Share what you have learned with loved ones or your circle of friends.

2. Can you create your very own red tent? Maybe it's having special red bed sheets, a red moon time journal, or a red candle; something that evokes this ancient tradition within you.

Chapter 3

---·—

PMS: A Female Curse?

PMS is a first signal that your body is telling you, 'I'm struggling here with estrogen issues.

—*Magdalena Wszelaki*

PMS is an acronym for Pre-Menstrual Syndrome. It varies from person to person, but generally can entail symptoms such as mood
swings, acne, refined carbohydrate and sugar cravings, irritability, exhaustion, bloating, low self-esteem, and anxiety; this list is by no means
exhaustive, and each woman's experience is quite unique!

PMS typically occurs during the Luteal phase—between ovulation and
menstruation. Exposure to chemical-laden products, stress-induced
cortisol roller coasters, and nutrient-deficient diets are among the most
common hormone disruptive triggers that women experience (more on
this in the next chapter). These triggers can cause higher levels of estrogen to be present during this phase, when in fact, it is progesterone that
should be greater in concentration.

One of the best things you can do for your body is to address the key
micronutrients that may have been compromised from years of exposure

to hormone disruptors. Then, find the foods that contain these micro-nutrients so that your body can naturally replenish its stores (you'll learn more about this in Chapter 5).

In this book, we will go over many of the common symptoms you experience, and what to do about them.

Two Options

In my experience, as well as the experience of my clients, many doctors only give women only two options to help with their PMS symptoms. First, of course, is the pill. The second option is other hormonal treatments to "cure" mood swings, to stop the pain, or to regulate the cycle.

The challenge with these external substances is that they disconnect us from our natural healing and cycle (period bleeding is only "breakthrough bleeding"). It stops us from accessing our inner well of power.

I recently had a conversation with one of my best and sweetest friends who was considering an intrauterine device (IUD) because of intense PMS symptoms, and not for any other reason. I don't blame her! Until recently, there has been very little education on what to do about those pesky PMS symptoms. Thankfully, we know there are ways to feel better by making lifestyle and nutritional changes. I will be giving my friend a copy of this book!

So, what if you don't have your period due to a hormonal IUD or the pill?

First and foremost, your own gut feeling, your own research, and your own health care needs are more important than anything I can teach you. So please, please do your due diligence.

My viewpoint is you do what is as natural as possible, meaning that you bleed prior to menopause. Birth control pills have done a wonderful job for the most part to prevent birth, though I do want you to know your options. In chapter 18 I will speak further about this.

Consider why you are experiencing the symptoms that you experience, and how to help yourself through them. If you are looking for birth control options, you may want to consider the copper IUD, condoms, the Fertility Awareness Method, and other more natural ways. After removing my copper IUD a year ago (at the time of writing), I feel much better. I'd love to hear your thoughts and experience with this!

Discussion Topics:

1. What are some of your PMS symptoms? Write down everything that you experience, from bloating, gas, acne, breast tenderness, and so on. Rate your current experience from one to five (five being the most frustrating) so that you can later compare it to your experience after implementing the knowledge and advice from this book.

2. Have you had a similar experience from your primary health care provider regarding birth control methods, or a way to help PMS symptoms?

3. What made you decide the type of contraceptive that you use? Was it convenience, research, or something else? Do you feel comfortable with what you are using?

Chapter 4

The Radiant Woman: What a Healthy Cycle Looks and Feels Like

What does health and beauty look and *feel* like to you?

Ladies, I think we can agree that we have been taught to think that *beauty* looks a certain way...and it's usually only one way! Particularly, we have been taught that beauty is an external quality that one is born with. The funny thing is that the "ideal" form of beauty is always changing.

On a recent trip to Rome, I *basked* inside of the museums and absorbed the beauty of the paintings of past eras. What I noticed was that the women portrayed in the paintings had soft bellies and breasts; quite unlike the models we see in the media and or Victoria's Secret shows today.

Growing up in the 90's, the idea of *heroin chic* (you can imagine what that means in terms of body type) was seen as beautiful and cool. I remember having posters of *Twiggy*, an icon at the time, as someone to look up to (not healthy for me). Today, it's the opposite! The point is that the ideal picture of beauty is always changing, and many women are looking to keep up with an ever changing ideal as to how they should or should not be.

At the height of my eating disorder (bulimia), I was the smallest and thinnest I had ever been, and I mentally not well. And yet, it was during this time that I was the most complimented on my appearance. Then when my father passed away, my mother lost a significant amount of weight because she did not have an appetite from the grief (my parents were deeply in love), and also began smoking a pack of cigarettes every few days to get by. During this unhealthy time in her life, she was also complimented left, right, and center on her weight and how good she looked (she was never a heavy set woman in the first place either). Strange, right?

Something was very, very wrong with this picture, which is why I am such an advocate for wellness from the inside out. How we look on the outside, does not always reflect health on the inside. Let's create sustainable beauty and vitality in *all* ways together.

Will you take a journey into redefining beauty with me?

I believe that when a woman is truly healthy from the inside out, she is stunningly beautiful.

Here are some beautiful and healthy qualities to work towards:

Physical

- Healthy, glowing skin. I am sure we can all agree that healthy skin is beautiful, and beautiful skin is healthy! Beautiful skin comes from eating healthy fats, consuming an abundance of vitamin-rich foods, drinking lots of water, and having a healthy digestion, healthy lungs, and more!

- Healthy, strong hair. Aside from certain genetic factors that play into hair loss, most of the time we can use our diet and lifestyle to achieve healthy and beautiful hair. Healthy hair results from having healthy circulation, eating high quality protein, balanced hormone levels, and consuming nourishing foods such as salmon, eggs, berries, and sweet potatoes.

- Healthy body composition. This does not refer to BMI, or what your scale tells you! I am not a fan of some of those tools either. This also isn't about looking a certain way or fitting an idea. For example, we now understand that excess cortisol (stress hormone) tends to accumulate in the abdomen. Excess estrogen (discussed more in the next chapter) is associated with an accumulation of fat in the hips and thighs. The more we achieve a healthy hormone profile, the more we will have a healthier body composition.

- A radiant smile. Who isn't absolutely stunning when they smile? Everyone is! Having healthy mouth and gut bacteria, through fibre and fermented foods make an enormous difference in our oral health, along with vitamins K, D, magnesium, calcium, phosphorus and more (Holistic Dental Care - Nadine Artemis is a great read for more information).

- Sound sleep. It differs from person to person to how much sleep you need (and it will change based on your cycle too!), though typically you want to aim for 6-9 hours of sleep per night, sleeping at the same time, and sleeping through the night. Please be sure to create a peaceful night time ritual for yourself.

- Elimination and digestion. If you suffer from even occasional bloating, gas or indigestion, please know that it doesn't have to be your norm. Eating should be a pleasurable experience for the mind, body and soul, and if you have any pain or discomfort, I encourage you to seek the help of a healthcare professional. As for elimination, I highly recommend looking up the Bristol Stool Chart to assess the health of your bowel movements. Not the sexiest conversation, but someone has to do it! This is a very important indicator of your health and should not be ignored or put off.

Emotional, Mental, Spiritual

- Balanced mood. If you find yourself shifting from different moods or having mood swings, it typically can indicate a blood sugar imbalance, excess estrogen, amino acid deficiency, and more. Please be sure to seek solutions.

- A purpose, vision and a goal. I believe that we each came here to fulfil a purpose that is unique to us, and that the soul communicates to us via the body to have us listen through symptoms (if we ignore the messages). My highest recommendation is that you take the time to paint a vision of the kind of life you would like to live, and work towards accomplishing that every single day for the rest of your life.

- Gratitude. When you are grateful for all that you have, all that you are, and all that has come before you, you will have a glow about you that radiates from the inside out. You will also feel more at peace and internally calm.

- Acceptance. This goes hand in hand with gratitude, and surrendering is a powerful ingredient in this recipe as well. When we accept the way things are and the way things are not, we have complete freedom. This is not to say that we accept concepts like slavery or racism; rather, this is looking first and foremost into our own lives and releasing the story that our boss should be nicer, that the weather needs to get warmer, etc. This means first accepting that this is the way that things currently are, then using self-responsibility to make appropriate changes.

- Self-responsibility. This is very important, and the most successful people that I know have a strong sense of self-responsibility. Self-responsibility means to embody the notion of, "If not now, when? If not me, who?" We must know that it is up to us to make the appropriate changes in our own lives and in the world (with help along the way). When we take 100% responsibility for every aspect of our lives, then can we have the power to change it. If we play the victim role and give away 20% of the responsibility to someone else, or to a circumstance, does that leave you feeling powerful? You choose who is in charge of making change. This is a muscle that we are all continuously developing.

- Forgiveness. I don't know if it's a Scorpio thing or a Selin thing, but I tend to hold grudges. And guess what, the grudges only affect me, and not the other person! There is a saying that goes, *refusing to forgive is like drinking poison and expecting the other person to die.* That's a pretty intense statement, but the truth of the matter is that forgiveness releases the tension in our own minds and hearts and allows us to let go. Ask yourself: *What did I learn from this situation? How has it made me better, wiser, and stronger?* I recommend the Hawaiian forgiveness prayer, "Ho'oponopono" (pronounced *Ho-oh-Po-no-Po-no*), to dive further into this concept of forgiveness.

- Curiosity. Curiosity and playfulness go hand in hand, and there is nothing more beautiful than childlike wonder and curiosity. It instantly makes us feel and look younger, and makes life so much more fascinating and wonderful. What are you curious about? What is that curious whisper inside telling you? Go follow it (yes, you will often fail, but that whisper of curiosity is like the cave that holds your treasure)!

- Purpose. This is a big one. A woman (or any person) who lives and works with purpose and intention is sooo sexy! They exude confidence in all that they do, and create a meaningful life. Have you defined your purpose? It can be anything, and it is your creation!

Now, on to menstruation! Now that we have named a few qualities of health and beauty, let's discover what a healthy and ideal period looks like.

Signs of a Healthy Period:

Please note that this is possible for you! You can have a painless period and enjoy your period. Aim to look for these signs:

- You experience little to no cramps (and at the very least, they are not debilitating!)
- Your mood is stable.
- You experience no breast tenderness.
- You have little to no acne along the jawline.
- You have cranberry red menstrual blood that changes to a bit brown towards the end (brown is caused by exposure to oxygen). Red is a normal, healthy period color. The red should be dark or vibrant, like a cranberry red or fruit punch. The consistency should be similar to maple syrup.
- You have little clotting. When period blood clots are similar in size to a golf ball or consistently around the size of a quarter, it's time to talk to your doctor. It may be an indication of a miscarriage or a uterine fibroid (small, non-cancerous growth inside the uterus).
- You do not leak out of your pads or tampons within the hour.
- You menstruate every 21-35 days with no spotting in between.
- You experience little-to-no bloating.
- You perhaps have lower energy and a desire to withdraw from the world, but not enough to be napping all day long.

When to See A Healthcare Provider

It's important to know what is normal for your period so you can tell when something is out of the ordinary and just not right. If you're experiencing any prolonged changes in your menstrual cycle or any of the following signs, reach out to your doctor:

- Bleeding between periods (Remember, it could simply be from excess cortisol. This will be covered in upcoming chapters. Try some dietary and lifestyle changes first).
- Significantly irregular cycles that vary in length; shorter than twenty-four days or longer than thirty-eight.
- No period for over three months.
- If you're pregnant and notice bleeding.
- If you've experienced menopause and are still bleeding.
- Unusual pain during your period.

The most important thing is to pay attention to your body and the patterns of variations in your period. Minor changes in period color and texture don't necessarily suggest a health problem, and only you know what is normal for your own body.

Discussion Topics:

1. What is your definition of health and beauty? What are five words that you would use to describe them?
2. Do you think you are healthy and beautiful? Why or why not?

Action Steps:

1. How can you feel more beautiful and healthier this week? What steps can you take to feel more beautiful and healthy?
2. Who is someone that you think is beautiful? Let them know you appreciate their inner and outer beauty by telling them!

Chapter 5

Estrogen: The Hormonal Key to Your Queendom

Let's face it, we love to look good!

I used to think that caring about how I looked and spending money on my external appearance was arrogant, selfish, and superficial. In a way, I am grateful for this opinion, as it led me to work on my mind first.

With that said, I am at a phase in my life where I realize that, as a woman, putting even the slightest effort, energy, and attention into my appearance or how I smell for example, makes me feel more confident and put together. What do you get when you have a woman who is proud of herself, and who is beautiful on the inside and out? An unstoppable woman, that's what! Look out world!

Whether it be lipstick, shampoo, or shoes that make you feel like a badass, I recommend buying the most eco-friendly and natural products possible. Not only for the sake of the environment, but for your hormones! Many common beauty products contain harmful chemicals that impact our endocrine system (hormones) without us even knowing it. Over time, something called estrogen dominance begins to happen.

Estrogen, in this case, regulates menstruation, hunger and satiety, and insulin sensitivity, metabolizes cholesterol, contributes to bone density, and more! Without it, you may end up with symptoms of premature menopause such vaginal dryness, hot flashes, moodiness, irregular periods, brain fog, and more. Many women experience these symptoms in excess if their hormones and adrenals are imbalanced to start with.

On the other hand, too much of a good thing causes biological chaos, in the case of high estrogen! Here is the golden nugget about PMS: *typically,* why you have PMS symptoms of bloating, mood swings, breast tenderness, and more, is from estrogen dominance. Again, this can be supported through your nutrition, mindset and lifestyle.

Estrogen dominance has also been linked to allergies, autoimmune disorders, breast cancer, uterine cancer, infertility, ovarian cysts, increased blood clotting, and is also associated with acceleration of the aging process. Hormonal cancers are associated with stored fat, which produces the most potent form of estrogen, estradiol. This type of harmful estrogen is more difficult for your body to detoxify, leading to more circulating estrogen and "bad" estrogen metabolites (which is why good elimination is so important!). Also, with some autoimmune conditions, high levels of estrogen can actually enhance the inflammatory response of the immune system (though this is not entirely a clear-cut challenge or solution).

Thankfully, hormone balance is what this book is about, and excess estrogen can be supported through lifestyle and nutrition. I've done it, my clients have, and so can you.

Symptoms of Estrogen Dominance

- Decreased sex drive.
- Irregular or otherwise abnormal menstrual periods.
- Bloating (water retention).
- Breast swelling and tenderness.

- Fibrocystic breasts.
- Headaches (especially premenstrually).
- Mood swings (most often irritability and depression).
- Weight or fat gain (particularly around the abdomen and hips).
- Cold hands and feet (a symptom of thyroid dysfunction).
- Hair loss.
- Thyroid dysfunction.
- Sluggish metabolism.
- Foggy thinking, memory loss.
- Fatigue.
- Trouble sleeping or insomnia.
- **PMS.**

Causes of Estrogen Dominance

- Excess body fat (greater than 28%).
- Too much stress, resulting in excess amounts of cortisol, insulin, and norepinephrine, which can lead to adrenal exhaustion and can also adversely affect overall hormonal balance.
- A low-fiber diet with excess refined carbohydrates that is deficient in nutrients and high-quality fats.
- Impaired immune function.
- Environmental agents (Xenoestrogens. More below).

What Are Xenoestrogens?

Xenoestrogens are a subcategory of an endocrine disruptor group that has specific estrogen-like effects. When xenoestrogens enter the body, they increase the total amount of estrogen resulting in estrogen dominance. Xenoestrogens are stored in fat cells. The buildup of xenoestrogens have been indicated in many conditions

How to Avoid Xenoestrogens

- Avoid pesticides, herbicides, and fungicides whenever possible.
- Choose organic, locally grown, and in-season foods.
- Buy hormone-free meats and dairy products to avoid hormones and pesticides.
- Reduce the use of plastics whenever possible.
- Do not microwave food in plastic containers.
- Avoid the use of plastic wrap to cover food for storing or microwaving.
- Store food using glass or ceramic containers whenever possible.
- Do not leave plastic containers, especially your drinking water, in the sun (if a plastic water container has been heated significantly, throw it away).
- Don't refill plastic water bottles.
- Avoid freezing water in plastic bottles to drink later.
- Use chemical-free, biodegradable laundry and household cleaning products.
- Choose chlorine-free products and unbleached paper products (i.e. tampons, menstrual pads, toilet paper, paper towel, or coffee filters).
- Use a chlorine filter on shower heads and filter your drinking water.
- Avoid creams and cosmetics that have toxic chemicals and estrogenic ingredients such as parabens and stearalkonium chloride (There are a lot of amazing natural beauty companies out there now!)
- Use naturally based fragrances, such as essential oils.
- Use chemical-free soaps and toothpastes.

Excess Estrogen and Stress

Note to the reader: if there is any segment of this book that is the most important, please let it be this one.

Women are courageous, intelligent, beautiful, and resilient; there is no doubt about that. Our endocrine (hormone system), on the other hand, is a bit more delicate and interconnected with the rest of our mind and body. Think of your endocrine system as an interconnected web.

Imbalances in one part of the web will affect another.

Then there is pregnenolone, which is considered the "mother of all hormones," and is used as a precursor for most of the steroid hormones in your body. If the way pregnenolone is used is thrown out of balance, other hormones will suffer.

In an ideal world where you have well-managed stress, your body's stress response is turned on only when needed. You have plenty of time with your parasympathetic nervous system, which is responsible for processes like reproduction, restorative functions, and digestion.

With the pace of our modern lives and the demand on women, stress response is often activated for extended periods. With chronic or unmanaged stress, the cortisol pathway is prioritized and your body favors channeling pregnenolone to use for cortisol production instead (meaning the body is favoring stress hormone production for our survival over reproduction and relaxation). This results in less pregnenolone being available for conversion to DHEA and other related sex hormones.

Symptoms of Pregnenolone Steal

Symptoms of Pregnenolone Steal and elevated cortisol can be broad and seem difficult to pinpoint, but may include:

- Weight gain. Research in female populations shows that elevated cortisol as a result of stress is higher in subjects with a high waist-to-hip ratio.

- Infertility. A study of infertile women undergoing IVF therapy found that the treatment group had higher levels of cortisol and prolactin than the fertile control group. I've noticed that clients with infertility have high stress levels, demanding schedules, and require better stress coping tools (whether they know it or not).

- Low libido. Women who experience chronic stress were found to have lower levels of genital arousal than the average stress group. The study indicated that both physical (salivary cortisol level) and psychological indicators were related to lower sexual arousal.

- Spotting. This is a major indicator of having low progesterone (which comes from pregnenolone). This is what was happening to me when I had two to four periods in a month. If you asked me if I was stressed at that time, I would have said no, but now looking back I definitely was. If you are spotting in between your periods, please be sure to address this immediately with the principles in the book. Vitamin B6 rich foods, magnesium, omega-3's, and stress management will help. I would love to help you with this if this as well.

So what do you do about it?

Unmanaged or unconscious stress, paired with a low fibre diet is what I see as the most common cases I see for the women that come to see me. What you can begin to do immediately is to incorporate more fibre into your diet. This is why I do not believe in 'low-carb' or 'keto' diets long term, as they are not always high in fibre. Enjoy plenty of whole and fibre-rich foods like apples, pears, chia seeds, flax seeds, quina, barley, brown rice, celery, asparagus, broccoli, cauliflower, and more for every meal. Yes, you heard that right! Be sure that every meal you eat has plenty of fibre, as you need fibre to help bulk your stool and help to eliminate excess estrogen. Next, address your stress response. This first and foremost begins in your mind as we had discussed earlier. If you do have hormone imbalance, for now you may choose to do less high intensity workouts, and instead have a gentler practice such as yoga, weight training, pilates and more until your beautiful body is back into balance. I highly recommend exploring meditation practice, yoga, massages, float tanks, or counseling. Pick one, and take action!

Action Items:

1. Do you suspect that you have symptoms of Pregnenolone Steal? What is one thing you will begin to do today or this week to ease your stress levels?

2. Do you use conventional or natural products? If natural, begin to switch out your shampoo, deodorant, soaps, makeup, perfume, and more.

Chapter 6

Nourishing Nutrients to Optimize Your Cycle

Due to the nature of our undernourished and overworked soil (our current agricultural system), we are not getting the same amount of nutrients through food as we once did. This is why many of the nutrients in our food today are quite depleted. We may require a high-quality supplement to make up for it. Additionally, many medications such as birth control, statins, and antidepressants can deplete important nutrients in our body.

If you are hoping to become pregnant but are currently on birth control, please give yourself at least six months to refuel your body to conceive a healthy baby.

Important Dietary Inclusions for a Healthy Menstrual Cycle

Magnesium

There is a reason women reach for dark chocolate during phase two of the menstrual cycle. Dark chocolate is rich in magnesium, which is a common deficiency among women. Magnesium is a nerve and muscle relaxant and can lower stress, anxiety, and improve the frequency of bowel movements, as well as reduce fluid retention, which causes bloating. Go ahead and enjoy dark chocolate to up your magnesium, just make sure it is at least 70% cacao (and that you can pronounce all of the ingredients!)

Vitamin E

Sweet potatoes and almonds are great dietary additions as they contain dense levels of Vitamin E. Vitamin E helps protect the body from inflammation (think less breast tenderness) and has other antioxidant benefits. Be sure to consume this in your luteal phase if you have tender breasts! You will notice the benefits right away.

Vitamin C

Vitamin C is one of the most powerful cleansers of excess estrogen. It is found in its highest quantities in dark leafy greens such as kale, spinach, and chard, as well as in citrus fruits.

B Vitamins

Sunflower seeds are not only a great source of selenium, but also of the powerhouse micronutrient Vitamin B6. This vitamin initiates the enhancement of progesterone in the body.

Calcium and Vitamin D

In several studies, calcium and Vitamin D have been found to facilitate both PMS symptoms and menstrual cramps. Plain yogurt, almonds, figs, and tofu are excellent calcium sources. You can fill up on Vitamin D with, for example, eggs and salmon. It is a basic necessary vitamin in our everyday life, but it's also an important vitamin for the treatment of PMS symptoms. Calcium is also a key supporter of hormonal acne, as well as fatigue and depression, which are often caused by excess estrogen.

Omega-3s

Omega-3 and other good fats are building blocks for hormones, and are shown to help with menstrual cramps (Science Direct). Salmon, chia seeds, and nuts contain omega-3.

Fiber

This is one of the most important in terms of helping you to feel better during your cycle.

Fibers keep the stomach in top condition and the digestive system operational. Many of the good fiber sources also contain vitamins B1 and B2, which have been shown to play a significant role in the prevention of PMS symptoms. They also help to bulk your stool and excrete excess estrogen.

Enjoy plenty of vegetables, fruits, and grains, such as avocados, pears, carrots, sweet potatoes, bananas, berries, chia seeds, nuts, seeds, brown rice, quinoa, amaranth, or steel cut oats to get enough fiber. Most complex carbohydrates have a good amount of fiber. Complex carbs are your BFF!

Power Foods For Your Period

Ancient Greek Physician Hippocrates, beautifully expressed: **Let food be thy medicine.** I believe he was right. Here are some a few foods foods to eat for your a healthy period (and you will learn more about what to eat for each cycle in Chapter 8):

Cruciferous Vegetables

Think of foods like arugula, kale, brussels sprouts, cabbage, and broccoli. Broccoli sprouts, in particular, are a great choice as they contain an active compound called *sulforaphane*, which supports liver detoxification. These veggies also contain a substance called DIM (or diindolylmethane), which also assists with liver detoxification (needed to help clear excess estrogen). Meal ideas: Using arugula as a base for your go-to salad or putting a handful of broccoli sprouts in a smoothie can help give your body the tools it needs to do its job. I also love adding frozen cauliflower in my smoothies in the summer (I live in a cold climate) for hormone health and a creamy texture. Give it a try!

Lentils, Red Meat and Liver

If you do eat meat, red meat can give you a boost if you have low energy before or during your period. When you're losing a lot of blood, your iron levels go down, and red meat can help bring them back up again. Seek out grass-fed beef when possible! Want an even better option? Believe it or not, organ meats are high in iron. Try liver, if you're brave enough! *Pâté*, anyone? Again, aim for grass-fed meats. Lentils are also very high in iron, and you can make a lentil burger or lentil masala soup for example. Pro tip: eat iron with vitamin C to increase absorption. I.E: steak with bell peppers, lentil with lemon juice.

Carrots

Carrots contain high amounts of Vitamin A, which helps with progesterone production, optimizing the ratio of progesterone to estrogen. Start eating a quarter-cup of raw carrots each day a few days before your period is supposed to begin. Shred it into your salads, or eat it as a snack with hummus.

Beets

Beets are hugely supportive for liver detoxification and are high in antioxidants and nutrients, betalains, and betaine, which aid in liver function. Ultimately, these help your body eliminate unnecessary estrogenic metabolites. Like carrots, they can be juiced, tossed into a smoothie, or added to a salad.

Bananas

Bananas are one of the best mood-boosting foods you can eat thanks to its high dose of vitamin B6 (which is an amazing vitamin for hormones in general). They're rich in potassium and magnesium, too, which can reduce water retention and bloat.

Avocados

Avocados help to relax and soothe muscles because of their omega-3, potassium and magnesium content. They also help with breast tenderness as they are rich in vitamin E! You can put them in a smoothie, in a sandwich, or top your soup!

Herbs and Supplements

These herbs are fantastic for hormone health! Please consult with your naturopath or herbalist before taking these herbs and supplements to help with your PMS:

- Ashwagandha
- Shatavari
- Chasteberry
- Vitex
- Raspberry leaf
- Turmeric.
- Luscious Living Women's Moon Tea – *coming soon!*

Recommended Supplements

Supplements are what they say they are: supplementary! Meaning, they are great as an *addition* to your healthy diet and lifestyle. Due to the nutrients being depleted in our soil today (from monocropping or not practicing crop rotation, etc.), our soil is deficient in the healthy bacteria and nutrients that are required to produce healthy plants, and the plants themselves then do not have the same amount of minerals as they once did.

I lived on four different organic farms in beautiful British Columbia, Canada and we would deliberately test and add nutrients to the soil. We also added fermented alfalfa for healthy bacteria! It's important to remember that a lot of work goes into organic food. Many farmers are intentional about the deficiencies and do their best to make up for it. That's why their food also tastes so good!

With all that said, I personally recommend that most people take supplements. I take them, and below are my favorite supplements for PMS. Always try to get the highest quality possible (the grocery store is not the best place):

- B-Complex. This may help with mood and irritability, breast tenderness, and bloating.

- Magnesium. Your BFF for cramp relief! I prefer a magnesium oil or spray, and epsom salt baths are also fantastic.

- Evening Primrose Oil. This is great for skin, and it may help with progesterone balance. It may also be helpful for hot flashes.

- Vitamin E. Take this during your Luteal phase. It will really help with breast tenderness!

- Omega-3's with B12. Women who took both of these experienced fewer menstrual pain (Science Direct). Also, Vitamin B-12 has been shown to lower homocysteine levels, which can cause inflammation as well.

- *Diindolylmethane*, or DIM. This may help with strong PMS symptoms, though speaking to a naturopath or someone like myself is advised before taking this.

The Full Circle

I recommend planning for your period ahead of time with a few go-to meals using the foods and nutrients above. You also have your sample meal guide and more information in your book bonus too!

Chapter 7

What to Eat During Each Phase of Your Cycle

Now that we talked about what to focus on for menstruation, in this chapter, we will dive into the key foods and focuses for each phase of your cycle. Remember, there is no need to be perfect with this, it is simply a guideline! Always listen to your own body.

Before we go into what to eat (which is an abundance of variety, flavors, and options) I want to make an important note: Any time I see women struggling with PMS symptoms, or even women with strong menopause symptoms, when they have cut out or greatly reduced:

- Conventional dairy (most cheeses, milk, yogurt, etc. from the grocery store).
- Gluten (found in wheat, rye, spelt, couscous, barley, couscous, etc.).
- Corn (found in most packaged foods) and soy (I still eat tempeh and organic, non-GMO soy from time to time).
- Refined sugar.

I won't go further into it than that, and I recommend you do your own research. Most of all, it's important to experiment.

I still eat high quality cheese (such as brie, camembert, or others) as well as regular pizza from time to time. But that is the key, *from time to time*. Moderation. I certainly do not believe in deprivation, so just be mindful of getting the highest quality possible! I live in Canada, and when I eat bread, even if it's sourdough bread from a local bakery, I still get acne on my forehead several days later. When I visit the U.S., I am bloated for the rest of the day after eating bread! In Italy, however, I ate bread and pasta daily and did not have a single issue (Italy and issues? Non possibile!). I attribute this to the soil quality, as mentioned earlier and partially that I was in a "bliss" response the whole time. The point is, when we have healthier soil, we have healthier plants, and don't need as many pesticides. Think of gut bacteria like soil bacteria; a healthy bacterial ground creates a healthy plant and body!

I often use avocado, hummus, cashew cheese, or pate to make up for the creamy feeling I would otherwise get from cheese when making a sandwich, for example. Nutritional yeast is also a delicious and nutritious alternative to a cheese-like taste.

PHASE 1: Bleed

Food Focus: Add nutrients; warmth, and comfort.

Day one of our cycle is the first day of menstruation. At the start of the cycle, our hormones are at their lowest as they work to shed the uterine lining. Because of this hormonal dip, energy levels are likely to be low. Support the body with plenty of filtered water and unprocessed, nutrient rich foods that keep energy and blood sugar levels steady. Focus on lean proteins, healthy fats, and complex carbohydrates such as root vegetables, wholegrain, and legume-packed stews.

For iron replenishment, try grass-fed beef, eggs, and fish, which are also a good source of heme iron.

Menstruation phase shopping list ideas:

- Sea vegetables, such as kelp.
- Sweet potato.
- Activated brown rice.
- Kefir or probiotic yogurts.
- Pumpkin seeds.
- Millet-based cereals.
- Wheat germ.
- Protein of choice: beef, chicken, lentils, fish, eggs, tofu.
- Nuts, supplements, and herbs.
- Magnesium.
- B Vitamins.

PHASE 2: Follicular

Food Focus: Keep it fresh! Add gut-friendly foods.

Hormone levels, while still low, are beginning to rise as your egg follicles mature in preparation for ovulation. This is a good time to incorporate light, fresh, and vibrant foods. These include salads and fermented foods such as kefir, probiotic yogurt, or sauerkraut, which support gut health and detoxification.

Follicular phase shopping list ideas:

- Salad vegetables.
- Flaxseeds.
- Avocado.
- Broccoli.
- Nuts/seed mix.
- Probiotic yogurt (or coconut yogurt!).

- Zucchini.
- Buckwheat.
- Salmon.
- Kefir.

PHASE 3: Ovulatory

Food Focus: Keep it light, fresh, and focus on the liver.

Hormone levels are rising, particularly estrogen, as it aids in the ovulation process. Excess estrogen can have a negative impact on our cycle, including breast tenderness and increased spots, so nutrients that support the liver to remove estrogen are good to include and are found in foods such as kale, broccoli, onions, garlic and radishes.

Ovulation phase shopping list ideas:

- Quinoa.
- Eggs.
- Kale.
- Radishes.
- Fruits: berries, citrus, papaya.

PHASE 4: Luteal

Food Focus: Curb cravings.

Hormone levels reach their peak as we approach menstruation, and many women experience PMS around this time. It is possible to help manage pre-period moods and discomforts through food choices.

If you experience swollen breasts and bloating, avoid foods high in salt as they can exacerbate the problem due to the anti-diuretic effects of salt on the body. This is also a good time of the month to cut down on caffeine and alcohol, as these stimulants can aggravate PMS, as well as trigger anxiety and mood shifts. Move away from these with alternatives like sparkling fruit water, herbal teas, or chicory root, or by swapping your morning latte for a caffeine free version.

Luteal phase shopping list ideas:

- Cauliflower.
- Cucumber (water retention).
- Squash.
- Caffeine-free herbal teas.
- Sesame seeds.
- Spinach.
- Brown rice.
- Protein of choice: tofu, chicken, lean meats, fish and seafood.
- Berries.
- Turmeric latte blend.
- Dark chocolate, supplements, and herbs.
- Vitamin E.
- B Complex.
- Evening Primrose oil.
- Magnesium (lots).

Obviously, these lists are not set in stone. Don't be too strict with it! Enjoy your experience, and seek out what works for your body!

Chapter 8

Invisible Friends and Hormone Balance

When we think of bugs, and bugs *living* in our bodies, most of us are grossed out, right? But these are the kind of bugs you want to have in your body! If they weren't there, you would actually be quite ill.

As you may have noticed from this book, every system in the body is connected, and our gut is intrinsically linked to our overall health and hormone balance.

Over the years, there has been an increasing amount of research between these invisible "friends" we call the *gut microbiome*. This refers specifically to the microorganisms living in your intestines. You may have 300 to 500 different species of bacteria in your digestive tract. This is good! Some microorganisms can be harmful to your health, but many are incredibly beneficial and even necessary for having a healthy body.

Optimizing our gut health is key to keeping our hormones in balance. Gut health is extremely important because the microbiome has many functions.

These include:

- Aiding the synthesis and regulation of hormones and feel good neurotransmitters.
- Facilitating the absorption of macro and micronutrients.
- Playing an important role in the immune system.
- Contributing to the regulation of estrogen levels in the body..

When the gut microbiome is healthy, the estrobolome (collection of bacteria in the gut that metabolizes the body's estrogen) helps to regulate estrogen levels. What happens to most people is, through years of antibiotic and medication use (including birth control), we may develop something called "gut dysbiosis," or in other words, an imbalance of bacteria in the body. This is when we begin to see mood challenges, digestion troubles, and more. I recommend listening to the interview on the Luscious Living podcast with Dr. Emeran Mayer, Best Selling Author of the Mind-Gut Connection, to learn more.

What feeds this good bacteria is fiber! Do you see how it comes full circle?

Signs of an Unhealthy Gut

There are many signs of an unhealthy gut. Here are a few:

- Digestive issues (bloating, gas, diarrhea or constipation).
- Weight changes.
- Food sensitivities.
- Fatigue.
- Skin irritation.
- Autoimmune conditions.
- Hormonal imbalance.

So, what can you do about it? Eat more fiber, and eat more fermented foods! Having a calm, balanced mind is also important. Seek therapy if you need it.

Here are my favorite fiber rich foods:

- Blackberries, blueberries, strawberries, cherries.
- Steel cut oats, quinoa, amaranth, millet, couscous, brown rice.
- Lentils, chickpeas, etc. (be sure to soak them).
- Avocados, carrots, tomatoes, cucumbers, turnips, potatoes, red cabbage, mushrooms, eggplant, zucchini, radish.
- Collard greens, broccoli, cauliflower, brussels sprouts.
- Pear, apples, banana, mango, papaya.
- Leeks, onions, garlic, Jerusalem artichoke.
- Chia seeds, flax seeds, hemp seeds.

As you can see, it is basically an example of whole foods.

Here are a list of probiotic foods to enjoy daily:

- Kimchi.
- Sauerkraut.
- Miso.
- Apple cider vinegar (get it "with the mother").
- Kombucha (I would have this in smaller amounts due to the sugar content).
- Kefir.
- Yogurt (I recommend coconut yogurt).
- Sourdough bread.
- Pickles.
- Olives.

Be sure to get things like sauerkraut and pickles from the refrigerated section of the grocery store, as the ones in the aisle have already been pasteurized and are missing healthy bacteria!

If you do not like the taste of these fermented foods, I recommend trying to get used to this taste profile. If that doesn't work for you, try using a probiotic (probiotics can be pricey, though they are great for travel).

Action Steps:

1. Pick one or two high-fiber foods that you will start to eat today. Look up new recipes and ways to incorporate this food into your everyday life.

2. Pick one to two probiotic rich foods and add them to a salad or a meal, and enjoy the benefits of this wonderful new habit!

Chapter 9

Seed Cycling: What's It All About?

Cycle syncing is a gentle way to support your body's natural rhythm using seeds such as sesame and sunflower seeds. Although there is not (yet) a lot of concrete research about seed cycling, some women swear by it! I personally do not use this myself, though have had some clients really enjoy it as a natural way to balance hormones. By boosting estrogen in the first phase and progesterone in the second phase, seed cycling may help relieve PMS, increase fertility, ease pain from conditions like ovarian cysts, endometriosis, and PCOS, and regulate irregular cycles.

How to Start Seed Cycling

Days 1-14: Menstruation to Ovulation

Estrogen levels start low from your menstruation, and steadily increase to prepare for ovulation. To keep estrogen levels in balance, cycle with flax seeds, as they contain phytoestrogens that adapt to the body's estrogen needs during this phase. If estrogen levels get too high, the lignans in the flaxseeds can bind to the excess so it can be eliminated from the body (so cool right?) Also cycle with pumpkin seeds, which are high in zinc to support progesterone production in the next phase. You can add these to smoothies, Buddha bowls, avocado toast, and more.

○ 1-2 tablespoons ground flax seeds per day

○ 1-2 tablespoons ground pumpkin seeds per day

Days 15-28: Ovulation to Menstruation

During this phase, cycle with sesame seeds, which are high in zinc and selenium and block excess estrogen; all essential for hormone balance. Cycle also with sunflower seeds, which are high in vitamin E to support progesterone levels.

○ 1-2 tablespoons ground sunflower seeds per day

○ 1-2 tablespoons ground sesame seeds per day

What if you don't have a 28-day menstrual cycle?

Don't worry! You can adjust the length of time you consume each seed combination based on your cycle length. This is why I highly recommend tracking your cycle.

What if you have an irregular or missing period?

No worries! You can use the concepts in this book to bring your cycle back to balance...and, it's possible to seed a cycle even if you have irregular or missing periods. Instead of rotating with the phases of your cycling, you'll follow the phases of the moon as a general guideline. In this case, day 1 of your cycle would begin with the new moon.

Days 1-14 (new moon to full moon), eat pumpkin seeds and flax seeds.

Days 15-28 (full moon to new moon), eat sunflower seeds and sesame seeds.

Sure, this may seem a little odd, but the moon is powerful! Have you ever noticed that the moon and the average menstrual cycle are both 28 days? This is no coincidence. Many women's cycles (when balanced) naturally follow the phases of the moon.

Chapter 10

Beat Bloating, Babe!

There is nothing more uncomfortable than feeling bloated, right? Not only is it difficult to concentrate when we are feeling bloated, but we also have to wear different clothes to hide how we look! So let's dive straight into it: how to get rid of period bloating!

Foods like bananas and dark leafy greens contain essential minerals, such as magnesium and potassium, that lessen water retention and bloating by countering with sodium in the body. The more salty foods you consume, the more likely it is that your body will retain water to counterbalance it. Reducing your intake of refined sugars is also an important step to reducing period bloating. Foods that are high in sugar encourage the pancreas to release a hormone called insulin, which, in high levels, causes water retention and period bloating.

To stop bloating before your period, follow these methods:

- Avoid salty foods to help decrease water retention in the body (i.e. chips, food from a box, fast food).
- Eat potassium-rich foods like bananas, cooked spinach, cooked broccoli, potatoes, sweet potatoes, and mushrooms.

- Eat more diuretic foods like spinach, asparagus, pineapples, cucumber, leeks, ginger, and garlic.
- Drink lots of filtered water.
- Avoid refined carbohydrates, as these cause an increase in blood sugar levels. Increased blood sugar levels result in a rise in insulin levels, causing kidneys to retain more sodium. Excessive sodium leads to more water retention, causing bloating.
- Exercise regularly for a minimum of thirty minutes at a time.

How do you get rid of bloating fast? Here are some tips:

- Sip some warm lemon water with a pinch of Celtic sea salt.
- Try a dash of cayenne pepper and turmeric in your food. These can stimulate digestion, relieving pressure and cramps, and easing gas.
- Drink coconut water.
- Drink ginger tea. Ginger provides relief from menstrual cramps that trigger bloating, and helps to stimulate digestion.
- Drink peppermint tea.
- Eat steamed asparagus, which is a natural diuretic.
- Eat spinach. Spinach alleviates belly bloat by pushing fiber through the digestive tract.
- Eat more fermented foods daily, such as kimchi and kefir. Skip kombucha for now, as it's high in sugar.
- Avoid canned beans.
- Do yoga poses for digestion (I love the YouTube videos "Yoga with Kassandra").

How do you get rid of bloating overnight?

- Take a bath with Epsom salt.
- Eat bananas, as they are rich in potassium, a nutrient that helps in the regulation of fluid balance to flatten belly bloat.
- Do not eat white onions, button mushrooms, raw spinach, artichokes, cauliflower, corn, broccoli, or kale.
- Avoid gum that contains artificial sweeteners and sugar alcohols like sorbitol and xylitol, which cause bloating.
- Pile on the cilantro to beat the bloat!
- Eat dark chocolate containing anti-inflammatory compounds.
- Eat slowly to avoid gulping air, which causes bloating.
- Drink lemon water.
- Avoid eating anything greasy.
- Work with me on restoring gut health. Book a call with me to learn more.

Action Steps:

1. Do you tend to feel bloated before your period? What is one thing you can reduce or eliminate from your diet or lifestyle to help reduce bloating?
2. Pick one of the suggestions listed above and practice it for this upcoming luteal phase!

Chapter 11

PMS and Headaches: Why?

The last thing you need during PMS is a headache. Would you be surprised to know that estrogen and headaches have a relationship?

Scientists are only now beginning to understand the role that estrogen and other sex hormones play when it comes to the body's ability to cope with both emotional and physical pain.

When estrogen levels are high, your brain responds quickly to pain. This releases a wave of endorphins that help your body minimize the sensations of both physical and emotional pain. When estrogen levels are lowered, a process that begins about a week before the first day of your period, your brain cannot combat pain as efficiently and effectively as it can during the rest of your cycle.

For some of us, this dip in estrogen can trigger menstrual headaches and migraines either before, during, or towards the end of our cycle.

Please refer back to Chapter 5 on Estrogen Dominance to become more familiar with this, and to understand how to clear excess estrogen from your beautiful body.

Chapter 12

Weight Gain and PMS: Great, Thanks!

If you're like me, you know that your cycle is coming soon because of how hungry you feel! Although I no longer experience pain, I still want to eat everything!

Here's what I do to avoid gaining weight during PMS (if that is your goal too):

- This is not the time to starve your body. Nourish yourself with a healthy and hearty and warm breakfast, lunch, and dinner. As you learned in previous chapters, please include more complex carbs, seaweeds, legumes, seeds and meat (if you're omnivorous). Examples include steel cut oats with blueberries and chia seeds, lentil masala soup, grass-fed beef chili, and roasted veggies.

- Reduce snacking throughout the day. This simple trick has single handedly helped me release over ten pounds. Eat substantially throughout the day and be sure to include protein with each meal, such as eggs, tempeh, tofu, nuts and seeds. Drinking a high-quality green or oolong tea helps me to also feel satiated.

- Track calories if you need to. This used to be a trigger for me, and I don't recommend it if this is something you struggle with. Yet, it can also be highly enlightening if you are open to it. I like free MyFitnessPal or LoseIt for free apps.

- Reduce liquid calories. It's easy to think that a matcha latte wouldn't be many calories and is therefore healthy, but the calories in the *latte* can add up! Aim for herbal teas, green tea, white tea, pu-erh tea, rooibos, or include alternatives to dairy milks to keep the calorie count low.

- Move more! Aim to move a minimum thirty minutes daily as it helps to activate something called *mTOR,* which helps you detoxify your body. On your cycle, remember to have a gentle practice but still keep moving, even if it's yoga or simply dancing in your kitchen, our beautiful bodies were meant to move!

- Pile your plate with your favorite non-starchy veggies such as spinach, kale, broccoli, cauliflower and more.Make them taste great! Search for brand new recipes and have fun with it.

- Enjoy what you want to enjoy. Make it pleasurable. Get a plate out. Slowly savor each bite of whatever you are eating. Aim for ingredients that you can pronounce, and please avoid high fructose corn syrup!

Chapter 13

Cramps: How to Deal

Ahhh … the million-dollar question. How can I get rid of those awful period cramps?

There is nothing more frustrating than period cramps! I remember a time when cramps used to wake me up at night. Some women are completely debilitated from period cramps and have to miss out on school or work. Whether your cramps are mild or deathly strong, using the useful tips and information in this book can help you begin to feel better.

Note: Menstrual cramps can be "primary" or "secondary." Primary *dysmenorrhea* (the clinical word for painful periods) is caused by the period itself. Secondary dysmenorrhea is period pain with a different root cause, such as a health condition like endometriosis. The following information is meant to help with primary dysmenorrhea.

So, what causes period cramps?

Menstrual cramps are likely caused by an excess of *prostaglandins*; these are hormone-like compounds that are released from the uterine lining (the endometrium) as it prepares to be shed. Prostaglandins help the uterus contract and relax, so that the endometrium can detach and flow out of your body. These physical actions taking place are a necessary part of the process.

However, in excess, they cause pain if the uterus contracts strongly, blood flow is reduced, and the supply of oxygen to the uterus muscle tissue decreases.

Inflammation may also play a role. People who experience more menstrual pain have also been shown to have higher levels of inflammatory markers in the blood, even after adjusting for factors related to chronic inflammation, like BMI, smoking, or alcohol consumption.

How can you relieve period cramps?

All methods of cramp relief do at least one of the following:

- Reduce inflammation.
- Limit prostaglandin production.
- Block pain.
- Increase uterine blood flow, or treat an underlying condition, like endometriosis.

Methods you might try include:

- Keep the body warm: heat packs, tea, soup, broth.
- Dietary changes (see previous chapters). Most importantly, reduce or eliminate dairy and gluten, and add omega-3's as they have been shown to be just as effective if not more, than pain killers (The National Center for Biotechnology Information).
- Supplementation, specifically magnesium and omega-3's for cramps (see Chapter 6).
- Stress relief: foam rolling, yin yoga, bath, massage, reflexology, acupuncture, float tank, etc.
- Quitting smoking.

- Exercise: yoga, pilates, and long walks during your cycle.
- Vaginal steaming - but not during your cycle (see Chapter 17).

It's not medically proven but here is a go to tip for cramps that I use and love:

On the first day of my period, I get a steaming hot bowl of Vietnamese pho. It relieves any discomfort instantly! Try it out!

Chapter 14

Banishing Hormonal Acne

So, you thought acne would end after your teenage years, right? There is nothing more frustrating than having acne as an adult.

There are many potions and creams that are marketed to women to "fight breakouts." While some of these may work, I have always had more success resolving adult acne through my diet. When I was a teen, I was on expensive three-step programs, which failed in resolving my acne. This chapter will focus on why you may still be experiencing acne as an adult.

Hormonal acne will usually appear along the chin and jawline (take a look at Chinese Face Mapping - you may notice an interesting connection with your acne troubles in connection to your other organs.) If you experience acne around PMS like clockwork, then read and understand the following tips:

- Find out which foods lead to an acne flair. Usually, dairy products can be the cause of acne around the jawline. Hormones such as prolactin, estrogens, progesterone, corticoids, and androgens are all commonly found in dairy. These elevated levels of hormones can lead to an increase in sebum production, causing acne.
- Clear excess estrogen (refer to Chapter 5).

- Limit alcohol. Alcohol is pro-inflammatory and can disrupt digestive health. It can also temporarily impair liver functions, impairing detoxification and causing acne.

- Get your fluids and fiber! Constipation can prevent the elimination of excessive hormone reserves. If you have issues with constipation, make sure you are drinking enough water. Aim to slowly increase your fiber intake, consume more healthy fats, and consider a probiotic (you are already eating fermented foods now, right?) *

- Reduce stress. This tip can be somewhat annoying because it's very common, but finding a form of mindfulness-based practice such as journaling, yoga, meditation, float tank, massage, reiki, etc., can be helpful in soothing the mind.

- Keep the kidneys clean and free of toxins by eating clean and boosting your intake of fruits, herbs and vegetables. Specifically eat more: parsley, basil, apple cider vinegar, kidney beans, dates, pomegranate, lemon juice, and dandelion root (you can consume this in a tea).

*A note on constipation:

I mentioned this earlier, but I again I need to say it again! Be sure to look up the Bristol Stool Chart online to get a sense of where your bowel movements are, and where they need to be. If you are chronically constipated (and I mean even a few times a week) I really need you to work on this. You'll want to incorporate lots of smart healthy fat sources including fatty fish like sardines and salmon, avocados, and olive oil , which lubricate the digestive system. Another constipation culprit is magnesium deficiency! You've heard me talk about this now... We don't eat enough of this underrated mineral, plus things like chronic stress, too much caffeine and sugar and toxic overload often deplete magnesium levels. Even if you eat plenty of magnesium-rich foods, again I recommend supplementing to get optimal levels. If you take too much, you will get loose stools. If that happens, back off a bit. Vitamin C is also great for your poop. Exercise is a great laxative too - a walk is great for so many reasons. Thank me later :)

These are the most important micronutrients for acne-prone skin:

- Zinc: Zinc has the most evidence showing a beneficial effect on acne.

- Vitamin D: You might have a deficiency if you live in a northern region or country. As a Canadian, I supplement with Vitamin D in the fall, winter, and spring!

- Vitamins A and E: Your skin will love you for these nutrients! I do not recommend supplementing with Vitamin A, as it is fat soluble (meaning you can't pee it out) and it's easy (and delicious) to get in food. For Vitamin A, go for eggs, carrots, sweet potatoes, butternut squash, cantaloupe, red bell peppers.

- Vitamin C: This vitamin has anti-inflammatory properties, and deficiencies in Vitamin C may result in more inflammatory acne lesions.

- Collagen: Collagen occurs naturally in the skin and I do recommend supplementing as it may help with skin elasticity, reduce visible wrinkles, and increase blood flow to the skin.

Chapter 15

The Two Forgotten Organs to Love

You or may not have considered the crucial role that your gallbladder plays in hormone health. I know I didn't! As a matter of fact, a poorly functioning gallbladder paves the way to PMS and hormone distress.

The Gallbladder and PMS

How is the gallbladder related to PMS?

1. The liver synthesizes bile. It packages up old hormones, including estrogen, as well as toxins that need to leave the body in the bile. It then ships the bile to the gallbladder.

2. The gallbladder stores bile and secretes it into the small intestine when we consume fatty foods. The bile breaks down the fat so we can absorb it, and the old hormones and toxins in the bile exit the body through the feces.

3. If your gallbladder is not functioning well, the bile becomes thick and stagnant in the gallbladder. As a result, the body reabsorbs the estrogen it should have eliminated, contributing to estrogen dominance.

4. To make matters worse, you can't properly digest fats with thick, stuck bile. The body needs to digest fats in order to synthesize hormones.

In a nutshell, poor gallbladder function may lead to the reabsorption of old estrogen, and a deficiency in the building blocks required for new hormones (The National Center for Biotechnology Information).

How do you support the gallbladder?

- Hydrate adequately.
- Avoid greasy foods.
- Include beneficial fats like cold-water fish, avocados, or hemp seeds.
- Increase fiber intake to 35/g per day.
- Check for food allergies.
- Consume more vitamins C and E.
- Aim for thirty minutes of exercise per day.

The Thyroid, Digestion and PMS

The connection between the thyroid gland and strong PMS symptoms is fascinating (or am I the only nerd here?)

Thyroid hormone stimulates the production of hydrochloric acid. Hydrochloric acid helps your body break down, digest, and absorb nutrients such as protein. It also eliminates bacteria and viruses in the stomach, protecting your body from infection. In relation to your thyroid, hydrochloric acid helps you absorb the nutrients needed by your thyroid in order to function, stimulates other digestive juices to start flowing, and defends against other unwanted toxins. If your thyroid hormones are low, hydrochloric acid will be low.

What can you do about it?

Step 1: Reset

I recommend trying to remove the following items as much as possible. In the beginning, try eliminating these foods:

- Alcohol.
- Caffeinated beverages.
- Dairy products.
- Items that contain gluten (such as wheat rye).
- Refined sugar is in artificial sweeteners (yes, chewing gum too).
- Nitrates found in processed fruit, hot dogs, lunch meat, and bacon.
- Carrageenan (found in many alternative dairy products).
- Deep-fried food, fast food and junk food.
- Partially hydrogenated oils, which can be found in many processed baked goods and snack food. These oils include margarine, canola oil, soy oil, peanut oil, and are often in packaged foods.

Step 2: Rebuild

- Fill your day with nutrient-dense beautiful whole fresh foods such as dark leafy greens, berries, nuts, seeds, and fruit.
- Increase the intake of saturated fats with extra virgin olive oil, butter from grass-fed cows, and lean grass-fed meat.
- Add high-fiber ingredients such as flaxseed, oatmeal, and chia seeds.
- Increase the intake of probiotics to restore the balance of intestinal flora. You can do this in a supplement, or with kimchi,

sauerkraut, kombucha, kefir, or pickles. Ensure you get the pickles and sauerkraut from the refrigerated section, as non-refrigerated options will be pasteurized.

- This may be one of the most important pieces of information I can offer: slow down your eating! If it normally takes you five to ten minutes to eat, try slowing your meal to ten to twenty minutes instead. Our senses help to increase hydrochloric acid and digest our food. If you have any sort of digestive troubles, please be sure that you slow down and begin to increase your desire to eat.

- Drink plenty of water in between meals, but not during meals. During meals, we can complete the necessary enzymes to digest our food.

- Supplement your diet with good quality digestive enzymes.

Step 3: Repair

- Take a high quality Omega-3 fish oil supplement.
- Eat slowly, deliberately, and with gratitude.
- Improve emotional health. Just as when you are embarrassed, your face flushes, or when you are angry, you might shake - anxiety, fear, depression and other emotional challenges symptoms can create physiological effects in the body (especially chronically) such as diarrhea, constipation, ulcers and gallstones. Taking steps to improve emotional health and promote a positive attitude can optimize the health of the digestive system.
- Include foods that help to repair the digestive and intestinal system, such as cacao, avocados, bone broth, butter, and more.

The Effect of Stress on Your Thyroid

When under constant or chronic stress, your body produces the stress hormone *cortisol*, your fight or flight hormone. If there's too much cortisol surging through your body, it can wreak havoc on your thyroid. Too much cortisol makes your thyroid gland work harder to produce enough thyroid hormone. This process can tax the thyroid gland and lead to imbalances of the thyroid hormone in your body.

I work with a lot of women, many of whom are mothers. Many are working mothers who tell me that they are not stressed, and yet their body language (and symptoms) tell a different story altogether...many of us are so used to being stressed that we don't even recognize how stressed we are!

Even regular thoughts such as: *I am not good enough. Is she prettier than me? Is she smarter than me? Ugh, my husband forgot to pick up the dry cleaning again!* can create stress and release cortisol in the body!

Stress and Hypothyroidism

The adrenal glands are responsible for secreting the stress-response regulating hormones cortisol, epinephrine, and norepinephrine. While these glands affect nearly every response in the body, when the adrenals are weak, they can cause symptoms of hypothyroidism. When you have a thyroid illness or imbalance, you are more likely to have inflammation in the body. This can lead to other diseases and health issues.

The "Should" Disease

Anytime we have a strong emotion, a physiological effect also takes place in the body. Do you remember the last time you were really embarrassed or angry? You may have had sweaty palms, your body temperature could have risen, or your hands might have shook. Remember, this all started with the *feeling* of being embarrassed...all of which is birthed from a *thought*. The thought of excitement, fear, and more, also begin this way. What's also happening in the body, is different hormones and neurotransmitters are firing off, or being shut off as we are experiencing any given emotion.

Left unchecked, chronic "negative" emotions (emotions that do not make us feel good and/or serve us) have chronic physiological effects on the body.

It is uncanny how often I see women who are judgemental very towards themselves (and sometimes of others),who have thyroid troubles. A common phrase in their dictionary is: should. "I should be further ahead. I should be at X weight. My kids should be X. My husband should be X."

What happens is that when cortisol chronically pumps into the body (from our thoughts of stress - *shoulding ourselves is very stressful!*) and it can shift the thyroid into a more inactive state, thus elevating reverse T3 levels rather than converting Free T4 to Free T3, resulting in symptoms of low thyroid syptoms. This lowered thyroid hormone is also important for glucose control, as it affects the number of insulin receptors available and how receptive they are to insulin. These symptoms of low thyroid can manifest as sluggishness, low energy or depression, difficulty losing weight, or hair loss, and sugar cravings to name a few.

The top nutrients needed for a healthy thyroid gland include:

- Iodine: This is an essential mineral that helps make the hormone T4, which is important for the metabolic process. It is a vital nutrient for growth development, energy production, and sensitivities.

- L-tyrosine: This is an amino acid that helps to regulate a variety of hormones produced by the thyroid, adrenal, and pituitary glands.

- Vitamin D: This helps to control overall thyroid production. Synthesize Vitamin D from sun exposure. If you live in the northern hemisphere, I recommend supplementing.

- Selenium: This is a mineral that helps to activate the enzymes needed to maintain normal thyroid function and stimulate thyroid hormone production.

Note: if you have high thyroid issues, please be sure to steam all cruciferous vegetables like cauliflower, broccoli, kale, and brussels sprouts in order to reduce their goitrogenic effect.

Here are the best foods for thyroid health:

- Oysters.
- Grass-fed beef.
- Brazil nuts.
- Eggs.
- Sardines.
- Spinach.
- Seaweed, such as wakame, nori, or arami. Another reason to eat more Sushi! You can also soak these beautiful seaweeds and add them to your salads, or to your soups as well.

Discussion Topics:

1. Are you someone who constantly "shoulds" herself or others? I find our struggle in our suffering comes from the perception that things should be a certain way when they are not. Ask yourself, what if I changed my perspective of the way things should be and accepted them, or tried to accept them, as they are? I know this might be difficult if you are experiencing deeply troubling circumstances that are out of your control, but I promise you that changing or altering your perception and eliminating the word "should" from your mental diet will increase your happiness and energy. Just try it for yourself.

2. If you would really like to better understand the areas where you tend to "should" yourself, begin to think about all the different categories of your life. These could include finances, career,

relationships, your family, your body, your health, etc. Think about all of the ways that you "should" yourself. Write them down.

3. Next, begin to upgrade your language. I encourage you to go from "I should" to "I get to. I choose to. I am discovering. I'm committed. I allow. I choose." Notice how you feel, and if you have a greater sense of power within you, discuss within your circle what you learned about yourself, and what you commit to replacing "should" with.

Chapter 16

What The Color of Your Period Can Tell You About Your Menstrual Health

We covered in an earlier chapter how the color cranberry red is a sign of health, but did you know that other colors of your menstruation can indicate other signs and symptoms?

Let's get into it.

At the beginning or end of your period, blood can be a dark red or shade of brown, and can have a thick consistency; it's normal for the first signs of your period to be bright red and thinner.

Bright Red Period Blood

Period flow typically becomes heavier on the second or third day of the cycle as the uterine lining sheds faster. This is the color you want your period to be!

Brown Period Blood

Blood first comes out red, and over time, it can darken to a brown color when exposed to oxygen. If your entire bleed is brown, you experience mid-cycle brown spotting, or you notice a significant amount of your period blood is brown, then this can signify low progesterone levels.

Pink Period Blood

"Spotting" is any bleeding that happens outside of your regular period. Some people experience spotting mid-cycle, also known as ovulation bleeding. Sometimes, pink menstrual blood may indicate low estrogen levels in the body. Some causes of low estrogen include being on hormonal birth control that doesn't contain estrogen, or perimenopause (the beginning of menopause). If neither of these are the case for you, please consult with your healthcare provider.

Gray Period Blood

If you have grayish discharge, this could be a sign of infection. If you experience heavy bleeding with pieces of grayish tissue, this could be a sign of a miscarriage. Seeing a healthcare provider is recommended in either situation.

Dark Blue or Purple Period Blood

If you're experiencing dark blue or purple bleeding, it means you have too much estrogen in your system. This just means you need to incorporate more fiber into your daily diet along with the other protocols and foods previously listed. So don't worry, you are in the right place and reading the right book (and again, please seek support when needed).

Orange Period Blood

Orange color, similar to a gray-red mix, may mean you have an infection. However, if this color is accompanied by a bad odor and severe pain, it could be a sign of an STD/STI infection.

Lochia

The bleeding that women experience for the first four to six weeks after delivering a baby is called *lochia*. This time is known as the postpartum period, or *puerperium*. It starts out relatively heavy, then from day four onward, lochia may be pinkish or brownish in color.

What about heavy or light periods?

If your period is light month after month, it could be an indication of a vitamin or nutrient deficiency, which could put your bones and heart at risk. Please refer to the earlier chapters for optimal nutrition, and consult with someone (like myself) to learn how to replenish those nutrients.

How do you know if you have a heavy period?

- A period lasting longer than seven days.
- Losing more than 80 mL of blood per cycle (or sixteen regular tampons or pads).
- Changing tampons or pads every hour or two.
- Needing to double up on period protection products.
- Having to wake up to change your tampon or pad throughout the night.
- Planning activities around your heavy period.
- Blood clots the size of a quarter or bigger.

What if you still experience a heavy flow after using birth control? Here is a probable answer that you have heard in this book: Estrogen Dominance!

Estrogen dominance is another one of the reasons why you may have a heavy period after stopping birth control. Estrogen dominance is when there is an imbalance between the amount of estrogen and progesterone released. When estrogen is substantially higher than progesterone, it becomes dominant. Heavy bleeding is caused by polyps, which are enlarged tissue growths in the endometrial cavity. Please go back to chapter 5 to help, and I highly recommend that you seek professional support.

Chapter 17

Vaginal Steaming
for Irregular Cycles

What the...*what?* Some of you may have heard of this, and some of you may be saying *"WTF"* right about now. Allow me to explain!

Vaginal steaming, also known as *V-steaming* or *yoni steaming*, is an age-old practice whereby a woman squats or sits over a container of steaming water containing herbs. The idea is to use the power of the steam and herbs to regulate the menstrual cycle. This has been practiced for centuries in Africa, Asia, and Central America (Birth Song Botanicals).

You may have heard that some women have experienced burns, but this happens only when not done properly. I find that most Western websites do not look warmly on vaginal steaming, but please do your own research, and please consult with someone who is certified, to walk you through this process.

Women who experience painful periods, periods that last more than four to five days, irregular discharge, fertility challenges, fibroids, ovarian cysts, and other issues have had significant and lasting changes with their cycle as a result of vaginal steaming (Garza et al.)

How does it work?

A vaginal steam carries medicinal plant oils to the vaginal tissue. These tissues are extremely absorbent, allowing the bloodstream to absorb these healing plant oils and carry them into the inner reproductive system. Once there, they aid the uterus in cleansing and repairing itself. Doing vaginal steams 1x the week before your period and 1x the week after your period can assist in relieving menstrual pain and reducing brown blood, thereby balancing menstrual issues over time.

Precautions / Contraindications

- Do not steam if you're pregnant or if you are trying to conceive; speak with a practitioner
- Do not steam during your period
- Do not steam if you have an IUD
- Do not steam if there is excess heat in the body due to fever, hot flashes, or night sweats
- Do not use essential oils, they are too harsh for the vagina. Stick with dried or fresh herbs
- Do not steam if you have any type of internal or external infection
- Speak with a midwife about steaming postpartum
- Speak with an herbalist or holistic practitioner if you are working to heal severe hormonal issues or infertility

Herbs to Use

You can find many brands and companies that have pre-packaged herbal blends that are specific to yoni steaming or you can buy your own herbs and create your own blends. Please consult with a professional, especially if you are dealing with specific issues.

How to Steam

Turn on some calming music, burn palo santo, or incense, and grab a book -plus anything else you'd like to add to make your experience enjoyable.

Ideally, you have a steaming stool (available on steamy chick, etsy, amazon). Alternatively, a large pot will do or a place where you can squat over the herbs without burning yourself. Please be very cautious not to touch the pot with your body.

It's often best to steep the herbs on the stove in 1 pot and then transfer them to another (cooled pot) for steaming.

Instructions

Start by boiling about 3 litres of filtered water. Once boiling, add 1 cup of dried herbs, reduce heat, cover, and simmer for about 5 minutes. Turn off the heat and let the mixture cool for 5 minutes. From there, you can transfer the herbs to a cool pot, place below your steam stool or pot, and get undressed from the waist down. Sit on your stool or toilet over the steam for 15-30 minutes. The steam should not feel too hot or aggressive. If it does, wait another 5 minutes & then try again. Use a towel to cover yourself and lock the steam in. Use this time for meditation, reading, or whatever feels right. When finished, discard the water and herbs in the garden or add them to your compost.

Discussion Topic:

Have you heard of vaginal steaming? Does it pique your curiosity? Why or why not?

Chapter 18

IUDs and the Pill:
What to Know To Glow

I n this day and age, we are certainly blessed to have an abundance of options when it comes to birth control: condoms, copper IUDs, hormonal IUDS, multiple options of the pill, etc.

While there are many benefits to these options—the prevention of pregnancy, decreasing acne in some women, and regulating the cycle for others—I do want to take the time to inform you of the risks as well.

For example, birth control pills may increase the risk of cardiovascular problems, such as blood clots, deep vein thrombosis (DVT), a clot in the lung, stroke, or even heart attack. Birth control pills have also been associated with an increase in blood pressure, benign liver tumors, and some types of cancer (Cleveland Clinic). Many women report extreme mood swings, depression, and weight gain from taking the pill (myself included) (Harvard Medical School). Please always do your own research.

Due to my natural loving nature (and terrible experience with multiple brands of birth control pills), I wanted to avoid anything hormone-based while remaining sexually active with my partner. I opted for the copper IUD. It worked wonders for me for about five years (though

I experienced significantly heavier periods and intense cramping compared to previous times), but I started to experience bleeding in between my cycles (I didn't realize it had to do with estrogen dominance). At one point, I had my cycle four times in one month! I was not happy, and definitely concerned! I had a gut feeling that I should have the IUD removed. While it did not help me with having two periods per month, I feel much, much better, and am glad I chose to listen to my gut.

Birth Control Pill Nutrient Depletions

If you are on the birth control pill, I want you to know that there are several nutritional depletions that accompany this, in particular, many B vitamins, including riboflavin, B6, B12, and folic acid. Birth control pills may also deplete vitamins C and E, as well the minerals magnesium, selenium, and zinc. The pill also inhibits ovulation, which is a sign of current and future health (US National Library of Medicine). Jerilynn Prior, Canadian endocrinology professor states that women benefit from 35 to 40 years of ovulatory cycles, not just for fertility but also to prevent osteoporosis, stroke, dementia, heart disease, and breast cancer. Also, compared to women who ovulate, women who take contraceptive drugs may have a greater chance of altered brain structure and a greater risk of depression and autoimmune disease. Please also be sure to feed your gut bacteria with pre and probiotics, as birth control pills can impact your gut bacteria. Probiotics produce beneficial bacteria – think apple cider vinegar, pickles, kefir, sauerkraut, kombucha or a supplement. Prebiotics then provide nutrition or food for that beneficial bacteria. Prebiotic foods include cacao powder, bananas, garlic, garlic, onions, leeks, asparagus and more.

If you are planning to conceive after coming off the pill, especially after being on the pill for several months or years, give yourself a minimum of six months before conceiving. The ideal timeline would be one to two years.

Copper IUDs contain, of course, high levels of copper, which can actually destroy Vitamin C in the body. It can also deplete zinc levels, lower iron, cause an unusual rise in Vitamin A, and aggravate B-vitamin metabolism.

It's important to note that estrogen and copper are related, as copper tends to raise estrogen in the body, and estrogen tends to cause copper to rise. Review Chapter 5 for more on Estrogen Dominance.

So, if you are taking any contraceptives, please make the appropriate dietary and lifestyle upgrades to be sure you are feeling your best on the inside out. Plan and target your meals and supplements accordingly! You may want to do a blood test to see where you are too. Consider using a more natural route for contraception.

Discussion Topics:

1. Are you currently using a IUD or birth control, and have been wanting to continue or switch out but maybe haven't had the time to start thinking about this?

2. Do you suspect that you might have an issue with your birth control or IUD? Might you need to start to consider other options?

3. If you are looking to conceive in the next year, what are some action steps that you can take to begin to nourish your body and bring it back to balance?

Chapter 19

Living a Luscious Life

When you think of living a luscious life, what comes to mind? We all have different ideas and preferences for self-care during our moon time. Here are a few of my favorite ways to take care of myself during my period:

- Yin yoga and long walks. I still love to move my body and find these two practices incredibly nourishing.
- Change your sheets, towels and underwear to red!
- Connect to different moon Goddesses throughout history such as Artemis (Greek) , IxChel (Mayan), Coyolxauhqui (Aztek), Maou (African) and more.
- Get more more sleep...Zzz…
- Track your cycle using an app or journal (I've been trying out the apps Clue, Femometer, MIA, and Natural Cycles).
- Watch a female centered movie or show (I will always love Sex and the City!)
- Rest. Menstruation is the natural time in the cycle for rest, so whatever you can do to settle your nervous system is going to support that. You could take a break (even for just a portion of your

bleed) from caffeine, alcohol, refined sugars, and even from social media, high intensity exercise, stressful situations, technology, or any other stimulants.

- Use reusable menstrual products such as a silicone menstrual cup, washable pads, or period undies. To me, it feels great to support mother nature while avoiding unnecessary chemicals and recurring costs.

- Eat warm and nourishing foods that support the liver, and the body's capacity for healing and renewal, such as vegetable and lentil soups, baked roast vegetables with brown rice, porridge with cinnamon and dates, as well as high-quality fats like avocado and coconut oil.

- Look into ovarian breathing from Mantak Chia (Taoist teacher).

- Connect with the water element. This could mean simply having a cleansing salty bath, enjoying a hot cup of herbal tea, or eating fresh, organic food to promote purification. Also, consider if there are areas of your life where you could be more flexible and fluid, or powerful, like water?

- Buy yourself flowers as you begin to bleed.

- Embrace the color red! You could light a red candle, wear a red flower in your hair, paint your nails red, or pop a red crystal in your bra.

- Connect with your inner Crone. Menstruation, being both the beginning and end of the cycle, is connected to our inner Crone—the wise, all-knowing woman within. A great question to journal on is, *what advice would my 85-year-old self have for me right now?*

- Ask for support. How could your partner, friends, or children help you during this time?

- Romance yourself! How can you make this a precious, sensual and sweet time for yourself?

- Dance! Slow and sensual, eyes closed, heart open; this is my favorite kind of movement at this time. Email me at hello@selinbilgin.com for sensual Spotify playlists!

Discussion Topics:

1. What are some of the ways in which you take care of yourself? (I would love to hear and see from you! Tag me on social media @_LusciousLiving_ with your favorite luscious lifestyle activity during your menstrual cycle!)

2. What is one thing from the list above that you will begin to incorporate in order to start nourishing yourself even more

Chapter 20

What's Next?

Well, you made it! We covered a lot of information, and I'd like to take a moment to recap a few key pieces together:

- If you are experiencing any PMS symptom, it is highly likely because you have excess estrogen, micronutrient deficiencies, dysbiosis, chronic stress, chronic alcohol intake, impaired liver function, xenoestrogens, hormonal contraception, growth hormone (from conventional animal products) inflammation.

- This can simply be cleared by drinking ample water, eating more cruciferous vegetables to help your liver function, eating fibre and probiotic rich foods daily, and healthy fats.

- Aim to use as natural products as possible for your makeup, skincare, shampoo, soap, laundry, and more!

- Reduce processed foods, processed sugar (even artificial sugar), conventional meat and dairy, gluten, soy and corn to see how you feel.

- Having a compelling vision for your life, and the beliefs to back up your desires will greatly increase the quality of your life. I recommend it to everyone.

- Prioritize spending time in nature, self-care, connection with other positive females, movement and sleep.
- You are beautiful, amazing and worthy. Thank you for reading this book.

That's a wrap!

Thank you for being the kind of woman who is always learning and growing.

I'd love to hear from you! If you have any questions or comments, please email me at hello@selinbilgin.com. Did you love the book? Share it with a friend!

Also, I invite you to participate in #PeriodPromise. Post a selfie on social media and use the hashtag #PeriodPromise…. What is your promise to your period? How will you begin to love and nurture yourself during this time? Let's be a part of the solution, together!

Please share what you have learned with your loved ones. The more empowered women we have in the world, the stronger, more beautiful world we will live in.

I look forward to hearing from you!

In love and service,

Selin Bilgin

Bibliography

Birth Song Botanicals. *Nourishing Herbal Remedies For Women And Children*, 2020, https://www.birthsongbotanicals.com/blogs/birth-song-blog/yoni-steaming-the-sacred-ori gin-how-to-steam-choosing-your-herbs. Accessed 10 01 2021.

Cleveland Clinic. "Yes, Your Birth Control Could Make You More Likely to Have a Blood Clot." *Cleveland Clinic*, 19 07 2019,

https://health.clevelandclinic.org/yes-your-birth-control-could-make-you-more-likely-to- have-a-blood-clot/. Accessed 10 01 2021.

Garza, K., et al. "Fourth Trimester Vaginal Steaming: A Foundational Study." *Fourth Trimester*

Vaginal Steam Study, 2019, www.fourthtrimestervaginalsteamstudy.com. Accessed 10 01 2021.

Harvard Medical School. "Can hormonal birth control trigger depression?" *Harvard Medical School*, Harvard Health,

https://www.health.harvard.edu/blog/can-hormonal-birth-control-trigger-depression-2016 101710514.

Health Link BC. "Basal Body Temperature (BBT) Charting." *Health Link BC*, May 2019, https://www.healthlinkbc.ca/health-topics/

hw202058#:~:text=Your%20body%20tempera　　　ture%20 dips%20a,C%20(98.6%C2%B0F). Accessed 10 01 2021.

The National Center for Biotechnology Information. "Comparison of the effect of fish oil and ibuprofen on treatment of severe pain in primary dysmenorrhea." *The National Center for Biotechnology Information*, 2011, https://www.ncbi.nlm.nih.gov/pmc/articles/ PMC3770499/. Accessed 10 01 2021.

The National Center for Biotechnology Information. "New insights into the molecular mechanisms underlying effects of estrogen on cholesterol gallstone formation." *The National Center for Biotechnology Information*, 2009, https://www.ncbi.nlm.nih.gov/pmc/ articles/PMC2756670/. Accessed 10 01 2021.

Prior, Dr. Jerilynn C. *Preventive Powers of Ovulation and Progesterone*. Centre for Menstrual Cycle and Ovulation Research., 2008. *Microsoft Word - Ovulation Series - Number 1 - What is Ovulation*, http://www. cemcor.ubc.ca/sites/default/files/uploads/1_What_is_Ovulation.pdf. Accessed 10 01 2021.

Science Direct. "Menstrual discomfort in Danish women reduced by dietary supplements of omega-3 PUFA and B12 (fish oil or seal oil capsules)." *Nutrition Research*, 2000. Accessed 10 01 2021.

US National Library of Medicine. "Ovulation, a sign of health." 2017, https://www.ncbi.nlm.nih.gov/pmc/articles/PMC5730019/. Accessed 10 01 2021.

About The Author

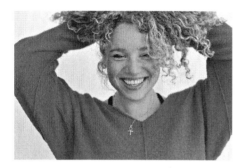

Selin Bilgin, B.A, C.H.N., is the founder of Luscious Living: Where Personal Growth Meets Wellness. She is a dynamic public speaker, wellness educator, and is certified in holistic nutrition.

Selin believes that lasting change, as well as radiance, vitality, and the ability to do the things we love in life come from having a growth mindset, inner alignment, and a wellness-centered lifestyle.

Growing up, the concept of "wellness" felt like light-years away for Selin. She experienced a background of yo-yo dieting, an eating disorder that nearly landed her in the hospital, anxiety (resulting in hyperhidrosis and insomnia), chronic acne, and hormone imbalance.

Selin now coaches women on how to find balance by regulating their hormones, shedding excess weight, and upgrading their mindset and lifestyle to go after what they want in life! She greatly emphasizes a mind/body/spirit approach to her work, and ultimately works with clients one-on-one in order to guide them back to their own innate wisdom and wellbeing.

Selin is also passionate about delivering wellness workshops to companies such as CIBC, RBC, Lindt, Gordon Food Services, First Capital, and many more.

Selin lives in Calgary, Alberta with her partner Eric, and loves drumming, improv acting and adding to her plant collection :)

Learn more about Selin at www.selinbilgin.com, or email hello@selinbilgin.com.

Printed in Great Britain
by Amazon

56199199R00064